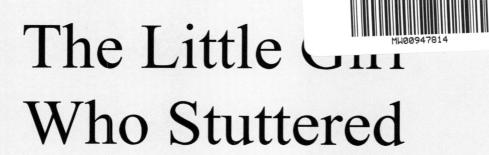

The Little Girl Who Stuttered

Written and Illustrated by Bernadine Stetzel

PRGOTT BOOKS Publishing

Norway, Maine

www.prgottbooks.net

The Little Girl Who Stuttered

Written and Illustrated by Bernadine Stetzel

Layout by Laura Ashton *laura.ashton@gitflorida.com*

ISBN 978-1537592558

Printed in the United States of America

PRGott Books Publishing

Dedicated To
Annie (castor) Glenn,
who has given sunshine
to many,
And whose rays have
shone on me,
I say, thank you,
thank you,
thank you.

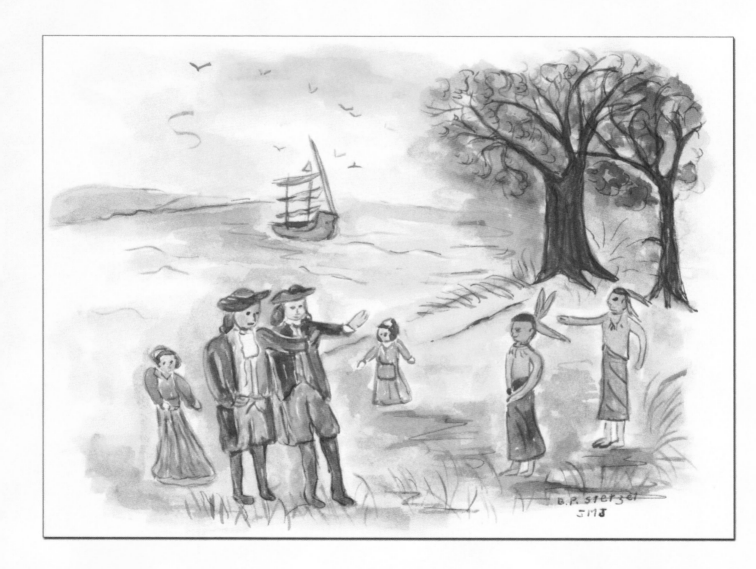

In the year of Our Lord, 1682, William Penn made his first voyage to the colony of Pennsylvania because of a grant of land in North America. It was payment for a debt that was owed to his father by the crown of England.

With several friends he sailed in September, 1682, for America and landed in October. He immediately began to work to establish the city of Philadelphia, and governed for two years.

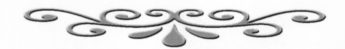

Penn learned of the persecution of his fellow Quakers and decided to go back to England to be of
assistance. In the year of Our
Lord, 1684, Penn made a trip to the
Netherlands to recruit men for his
second voyage to America.

While recruiting, Penn happened to meet a German by the name of
(Paulus Küster) who was visiting
there. Penn asked him if he was interested in going to America
with him.

He agreed, so Paulus left with his wife, Gertrude, and their three sons, Hermanus, Arnold, Johannes. They set sail in 1684 for America.

The (Küster) family lived outside of Philadelphia on land Paulus had purchased. There the (Küster) family toiled and suffered all the hardships of early pioneer life and reared several more children.

This family still survives today, living their strong heritage of courage, bearing crosses and achievements,

and continuing these is a little girl
named Annie. She was born February 17, 1920 in Columbus, Ohio,
to Homer and Margaret Castor, while her
father was in his last year of dental school.
This beautiful newborn baby never realized the strength and faith it would
take to endure trials that lay ahead
for her.

B.R. Stetzel
JMS

A year later, the family moved to New Concord, where her father set up his dentistry practice. New Concord was dubbed "Saints Rest" and Annie was to learn the true meaning of this title throughout her childhood. For her parents, sister, friends, church members all understood her and helped her to gain strength and courage to endure her handicap.

   Annie's speech problem began when she was three years old. At Halloween time, children came to the door with scary masks on for "Tricks or Treats". When Annie opened the door, being a sensitive child, she was frightened so severely that she became hysterical.

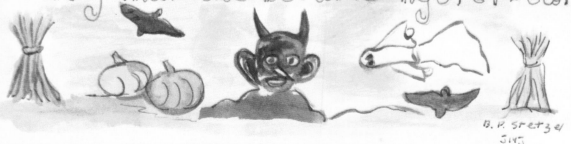

B. R. Sretzel
JMJ

Shortly after this, her mother began to notice a change in Annie's speech.

This little girl never let her handicap keep her from living a fulfilled life. She knew her limits as far as her speech was concerned, but this never kept her from accomplishing many other achievements, where she had no limits.

In school, her teachers avoided putting Annie in a position to emphasize her handicap.

instead they helped direct Annie to excell in the other talents God had given her.

These were many. Annie played piano, trombone, and she could use her speech clearly while singing. Sewing was another talent she possessed. Annie played many sports, tennis being her favorite.

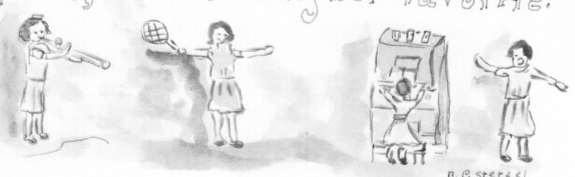

B. P. Stergel
5/15

When Annie became old enough to use the phone and receive phone calls, her sister, Jane, who has always been a very loving and caring sister, came to her aid. Her younger sister, Jane, received and made Annie's phone calls and relayed them to Annie and returned a message to the caller when necessary. Her sister was to play an important part in her childhood by assisting her in moments when she was unable to communicate.

When Annie was interested in trombone, she played in the town band with her sister Jane. A young trumpeter came into her life, whom she was to fall in love with in high school and later marry.

This young man was John Glenn. His father and mother, John Sr. and Clara Glenn, were friends

B.P.Stetzel
5th J

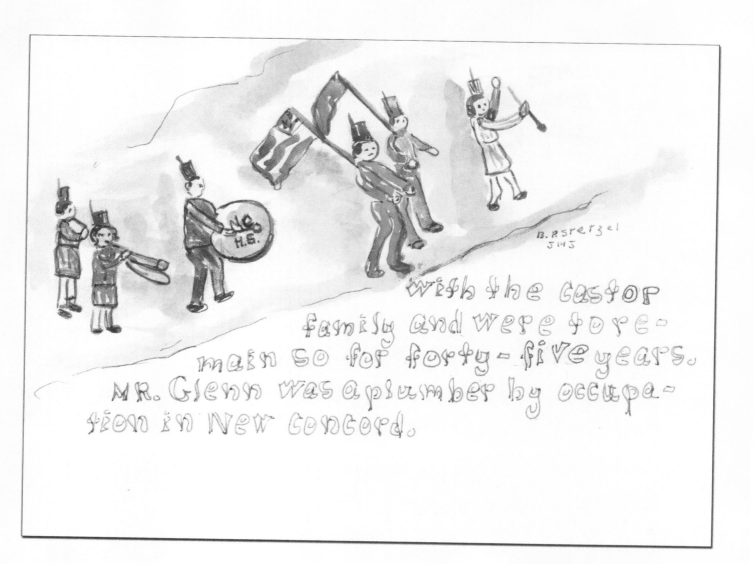

with the Castor family and were to remain so for forty-five years. Mr. Glenn was a plumber by occupation in New Concord.

Annie and John enjoyed many activities together. John also had a gift for singing. So many delightful hours were spent harmonizing with Annie and her sister, Jane.

During Annie's high school years, Jane was assisted by John in helping Annie in difficult times. During these trying years, her father and mother never stopped trying to find help for her speech handicap.

Annie and her parents traveled to Columbus, Ohio and Miami,

university to no avail. The doctors were puzzled and failed to find a reason for her problem.

Throughout her childhood, Annie was aware that not all children are kind, and some would make unkind remarks behind her back.

Sometimes, Annie accidentally overheard them. Of course, she was hurt, but she never, ever went home crying, asking for sympathy, but simply put these

remarks out of her mind, and became busy with positive activities.

This was a little girl with unlimited energy, talent, and courage.

Annie and John became interested in each other when Annie was a freshman and John was in the eighth grade.

Throughout their high school years, Annie and John attended many social functions together. During these years many phone calls were from John. They did not present a problem for Annie, because, for some unknown reason, she was able to speak continuously and distinctly to John. He was the only one she was able to do this with.

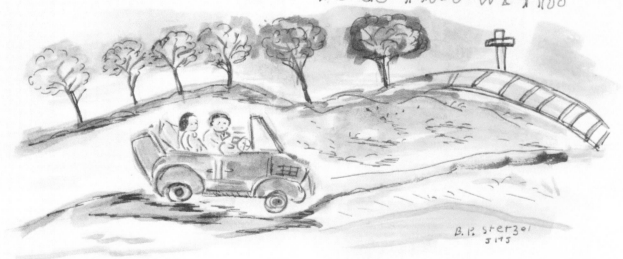

B. P. Sterzel
5-95

In high school, Annie became expert in secretarial skills, such as typing. Besides being very accomplished in these subjects, which consumed much of her days, she still found time to do volunteer work for needy organizations and other needy individuals.

Annie and John both attended Muskingum College. There were many memorable, carefree times during these years.

On the lake near the campus, Annie and John enjoyed ice skating on crisp, cold, snowy, moon light nights. They also enjoyed many other sports and activities, but they did not fail to realize the main reason they were there, which was a college education.

They both achieved high grades, And were well received by their peers.

In 1943, John and Annie were married. Shortly afterwards, John joined the Marine air force, and became a pilot. Annie was left temporarily behind until John was finished with his training.

War had broken out, and this was the first of twenty-three moves that Annie was to make in twenty years. Each time she had to arrange for all the packing and moving by herself, because John was on duty in many different parts of the world.

Annie spent many hours working for organizations that contributed to helping the soldiers over seas.

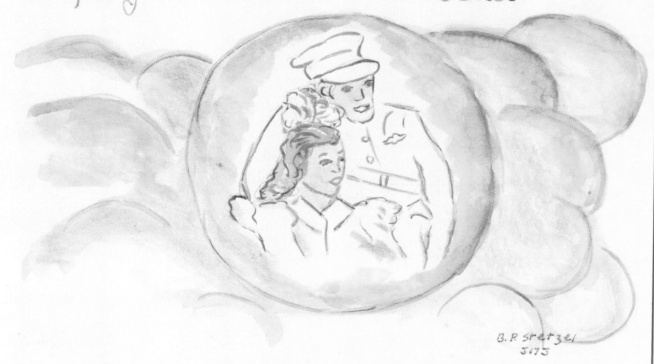

B. P. Sretzel
5-13

These were trying times, since Annie wasn't in "Saints Rest," where she would have immediate help. This situation would have been difficult for anyone even in normal circumstances.

Annie met this challenge with her usual strength and confidence that she could achieve it. In fact she enjoyed her duties and obligations and still found time to volunteer many hours for the war effort.

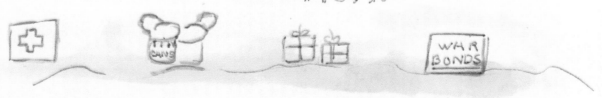

During these hectic years, Annie was to bear two children, David and Lyn. Even though Annie was alone with the children a great deal during these years, they were an enjoyment and comfort to her.

Every time the Glenns moved Annie made good friends with several people, whom she could rely on in emergencies.

One such incident, when she needed emergency help, was when Lyn punctured her foot with a rusty

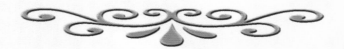

nail. Annie, failing to realize the severity of the puncture, passed the nail out, causing the wound to bleed profusely.

A neighbor came to her rescue when Annie ran to her with the child.

These twenty years were very stressful for Annie as she also worried about John's safety.

His first few years were as a fighter pilot for the united state marines, and he made 149 missions as a fighter pilot over south Pacific and Korea.

The most stressful time of all was when John was an astronaut orbiting the earth. This project was delayed six times before the mission actually occurred.

To alleviate some of the stress to the family, John told them at dinners and holiday get-togethers, the information he was allowed to pass along. He said everything was well calculated and had a back-up system in case of failure.

This helped Annie, but fear of failure was not completely relieved. It was the first time she felt in her heart that John may not return.

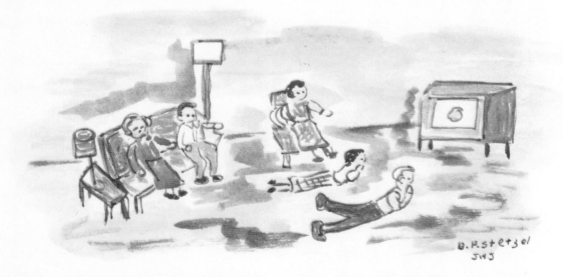

On February 20, 1962, Annie sat glued to the television set with only her children and parents present, as she wanted it, when John circled the earth.

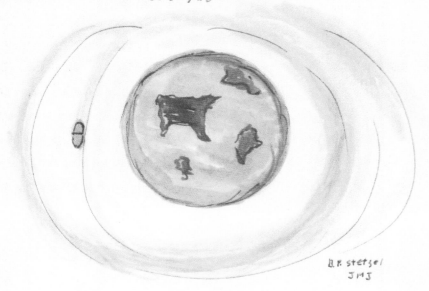

B.R. Stetzel
JMJ

Annie was very elated at this, as the whole world was.

John was given a ticker tape parade down Fifth Avenue in New York. During that ride, Annie was to share with him his success, as John would not have wanted it otherwise.

B.P. Stetzel
JMJ

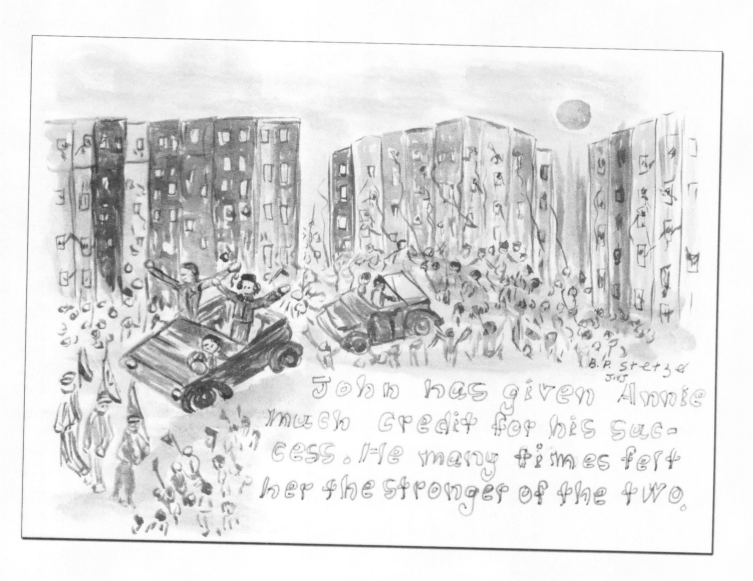

John has given Annie much credit for his success. He many times felt her the stronger of the two.

Over these 20 years, Annie had many good memories of John, her children, other relatives, and friends at holidays and other intimate times.

After John retired from the service, John and Annie were to lead a more public life. He became a consultant for the National Aeronautics and Space Administration (NASA).

They returned to Columbus, and John became an executive with Royal Crown International.

John again became interested in serving his country, and he decided to run for a seat in the United States Senate from Ohio in 1968. Because of an injury in a fall, he had to withdraw from the race.

Regaining his health, John ran successfully in 1974. During this time of campaigning, Annie's endurance was again put to a test. Many reporters and political people were not aware of her speech problem. Annie was criticized as being aloof, unfriendly and uninterested.

Since Annie was in the public's eye more than before, she was still searching for a doctor to help with her speech problem.

Early one morning in 1992, her search came to an end. Her sister, Jane, was listening to the TV and heard this doctor tell about his school for people with speech problems.

Jane immediately thought of Annie and listened very intently to each

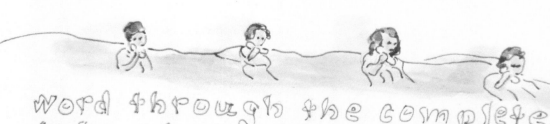

word through the complete interview. She went immediately to the phone to call Annie. Jane wanted to relay the message that this doctor had told of his many, almost miraculous successes using his new methods of treatment.

Jane was unable to contact Annie that day, because Annie's phone was constantly busy.

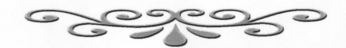

The next day, when Jane finally got through, she found the reason that the phone was so busy was because the many friends Annie had throughout the whole country were trying to contact her also in hope that this doctor could help Annie.

In January of 1973, Annie attended Hollins College in Roanoke, Virginia, with much success. She practiced a great deal during these months. On Memories Day, 1973, at Chagrin

Falls, Ohio, in front of the civil war obelisk, Judge William Thomas introduced Annie to speak in behalf of her husband, who was speaking at another ceremony elsewhere. The Judge was unaware this would be a first for her, but many people in the crowed knew of it.

   Annie stood in silence for a few seconds and wondered if she could do it. She had never publicly made a

speech before. With her usual courage and determination, Annie decided this would be a golden opportunity to try, and try she did.

The speech was such a success, that people who knew of her problem stood in tears. They knew what it meant to overcome this handicap that had plagued her all her life.

William Penn, the man who brought Annie's forefathers to America, brought to mind for Annie the first book he wrote during his religious persecution, "No Cross, No Glory."

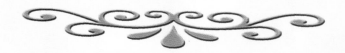

This was a great victory for Annie that she had finally overcome her handicaps one of the greatest being, When she went into a store. Now there was no more feeling of frustration over clerks thinking her also deaf and not having to write every thing down on paper.

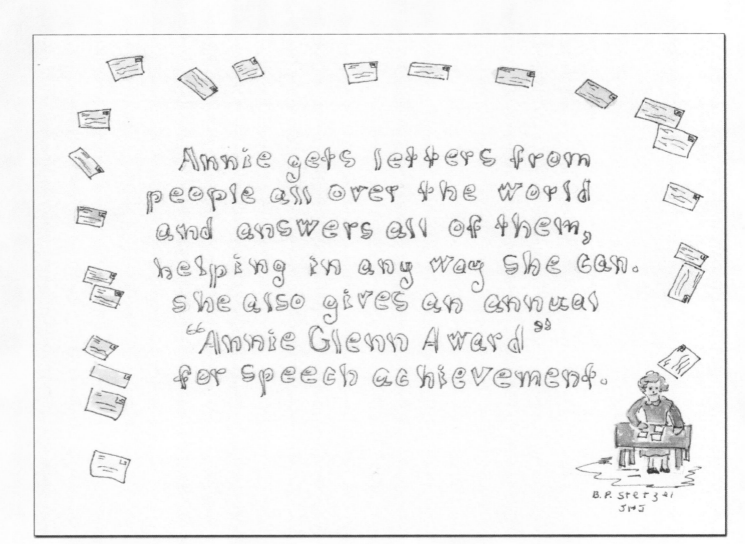

Annie gets letters from people all over the world and answers all of them, helping in any way she can. She also gives an annual "Annie Glenn Award" for speech achievement.

B.P. Sterzel
JMJ

Annie goes onto make speeches throughout many states, some are political and others are to speak about how she overcame her handicap. No one else was more elated over Annie's success in overcoming her problem than John. He had many agonizing thoughts about her handicap.

One morning, a young reporter found John sitting in tears in his office. The reporter asked John what was wrong, and John then proceeded to tell him that he was listening to Annie's very fluent tapes. He told the reporter that this relieved him of all the years of anxiety he had suffered.

Years later when John was being interviewed as one of the "Top Ten Persons Of The Year" in America, he was asked who was the bravest person he ever knew, and without hesitating John replied, "Annie!"

To handicapped children everywhere.
Let this story be an inspiration to sing out, "I shall over come!"
Then you too will be able to sing, as Annie, "I have over come!"

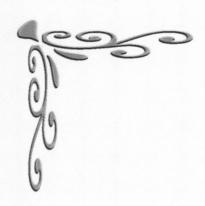

Dedication

Annie (Castor) Glenn,
who has given sunshine to many,
and whose rays have shone on me,
I say, thank you, thank you, thank you.

The Little Girl Who Stuttered

Corresponding
Page (P) Numbers

P 5

In the year of our Lord, 1682, William Penn made his first voyage to the colony of Pennsylvania, because of a grant of land in North America. It was payment for a debt that was owed to his father by the Crown of England.

With several friends he sailed in September, 1682, for America and landed in October. He immediately began to work to establish the city of Philadelphia, and governed for two years.

P 6

Penn learned of the persecution of his fellow Quakers and decided to go back to England to be of assistance. In the year of our Lord, 1684, Penn made a trip to the Netherlands to recruit men for his second voyage to America.

While recruiting, Penn happened to meet a German by the name of Paulus Küster, who was visiting there. Penn asked him if he was interested in going to America with him.

P 7-8

He agreed, so Paulus left with his wife, Gertrude, and their three sons, Hermanus, Arnold, Johannes. They set sail in 1684 for America.

The Küster family lived outside of Philadelphia on land Paulus had purchased. There the Küster family toiled and suffered all the hardships of early pioneer life and reared several more children.

This family still survives today, living their strong heritage of courage, bearing crosses and achievements, and continuing these is a little girl named Annie. She was born February 17, 1920, in Columbus, Ohio, to Homer and Margaret Castor, while her father was in his last year of dental school. This beautiful newborn baby never realized the strength and faith it would take to endure trials that lay ahead for her.

P 9-10

A year later, the family moved to New Concord, where her father set up his dentistry practice. New Concord was dubbed "Saints Rest," and Annie was to learn the true meaning of this title throughout her childhood. For her parents, sister, friends, church members all understood her and helped her to gain strength and courage to endure her handicap.

Annie's speech problem began when she was three years old. At Halloween time, children came to the door with scary masks on for "Tricks or Treats." When Annie opened the door, being a sensitive child, she was frightened so severely that she became hysterical.

P 11-12

Shortly after this, her mother began to notice a change in Annie's speech.

This little girl never let her handicap keep her from living a fulfilled life. She knew her limits as far as her speech was concerned, but this never kept her from accomplishing many other achievements, where she had no limits.

In school, her teachers avoided putting Annie in a position to emphasize her handicap. Instead they helped direct Annie to excel in the other talents God had given her.

These were many. Annie played piano, trombone, and she could use her speech clearly while singing. Sewing was another talent she possessed. Annie played many sports, tennis being her favorite.

P 13

When Annie became old enough to use the phone and receive phone calls, her sister, Jane, who has always been a very caring and loving sister, came to her aid. Her younger sister, Jane, received and made Annie's phone calls and relayed them to Annie and returned a message to the caller when necessary. Her sister was to play an important part in her childhood by assisting her in moments when she was unable to communicate.

P 14-15

When Annie was interested in trombone, she played in the town band with her sister, Jane. A young trumpeter came into her life, whom she was to fall in love with in high school and later marry. This young man was John Glenn. His father and mother, John Sr. and Clara Glenn, were friends with the Castor family and were to remain so for forty-five years. Mr. Glenn was a plumber by occupation in New Concord.

P 16-19

Annie and John enjoyed many activities together. John also had a gift for singing. So many delightful hours were spent harmonizing with Annie and her sister, Jane.

During Annie's high school years, Jane was assisted by John in helping Annie in difficult times. During these trying years, her father and mother never stopped trying to find help for her speech handicap.

Annie and her parents traveled to Columbus, Ohio and Miami University to no avail. The doctors were puzzled and failed to find a reason for her problem.

Throughout her childhood, Annie was aware that not all children are kind, and some would make unkind remarks behind her back.

Sometimes, Annie accidentally overheard them. Of course, she was hurt, but she never, ever went home crying, asking for sympathy, but simply put these remarks out of her mind, and became busy with positive activities.

This was a little girl with unlimited energy, talent, and courage.

Annie and John became interested in each other when Annie was a freshman and John was in the eighth grade.

Throughout their high school years, Annie and John attended many social functions together. During these years many phone calls were from John. They did not present a problem for Annie, because, for some unknown reason, she was able to speak continuously and distinctly to John. He was the only one she was able to do this with.

P 20

In high school, Annie became expert in secretarial skills, such as typing. Besides being very accomplished in these subjects, which consumed much of her days, she still found time to do volunteer work for needy organizations and other needy individuals.

Annie and John both attended Muskingum College. There were many memorable, carefree times during these years.

P 21

On the lake near the campus, Annie and John enjoyed ice skating on crisp, cold, snowy, moonlight nights. They also enjoyed many other sports and activities, but they did not fail to realize the main reason they were there, which was a college education.

They both achieved high grades, and were well received by their peers.

P 22

In 1943, John and Annie were married. Shortly afterwards, John joined the Marine Air Force, and became a pilot. Annie was left temporarily behind until John was finished with his training.

War had broken out, and this was the first of twenty-three moves that Annie was to make in twenty years. Each time she had to arrange for all the packing and moving by herself, because John was on duty in many different parts of the world.

P 23

Annie spent many hours working for organizations that contributed to helping the soldiers overseas.

P 24

These were trying times, since Annie wasn't in "Saints Rest," where she would have immediate help. This situation would have been difficult for anyone even in normal circumstances.

Annie met this challenge with her usual strength and confidence that she could achieve it. In fact she enjoyed her duties and obligations and still found time to volunteer many hours for the war effort.

P 25-28

During these hectic years, Annie was to bear two children, David and Lyn. Even though Annie was alone with the children a great deal during these years, they were an enjoyment and comfort to her.

Every time the Glenns moved, Annie made good friends with several people whom she could rely on in emergencies.

One such incident, when she needed emergency help, was when Lyn punctured her foot with a rusty nail. Annie, failing to realize the severity of the puncture, pulled the nail out, causing the wound to bleed profusely.

A neighbor came to her rescue when Annie ran to her with the child.

These twenty years were very stressful for Annie as she also worried about John's safety.

His first few years were as a fighter pilot for the United States Marines, and he made 149 missions as a fighter pilot over South Pacific and Korea.

The most stressful time of all was when John was an astronaut orbiting the earth. This project was delayed six times before the mission actually occurred.

To alleviate some of the stress to the family, John told them at dinners and holiday get-togethers, the information he was allowed to pass along. He said everything was well calculated and had a back-up system in case of failure.

This helped Annie, but fear of failure was not completely relieved. It was the first time she felt in her heart that John may not return.

P 29

On February 20, 1962, Annie sat glued to the television set with only her children and parents present, as she wanted it, when John circled the earth.

P 30

Annie was very elated at this, as the whole world was.

John was given a ticker tape parade down Fifth Avenue in New York. During that ride, Annie was to share with him his success, as John would not have wanted it otherwise.

P 31

John has given Annie much credit for his success. He many times felt her the stronger of the two.

P 32

Over these 20 years, Annie had many good memories of John, her children, other relatives, and friends at holidays and other intimate times.

After John retired from the service, John and Annie were to lead a more public life. He became a consultant for the National Aeronautics and Space Administration (NASA).

They returned to Columbus, and John became an executive with Royal Crown International.

P 33

John again became interested in serving his country, and he decided to run for a seat in the United States Senate from Ohio in 1968. Because of an injury in a fall, he had to withdraw from the race.

Regaining his health, John ran successfully in 1974. During this time of campaigning, Annie's endurance was again put to a test. Many reporters and political people were not aware of her speech problem. Annie was criticized as being aloof, unfriendly and uninterested.

P 34-35

Since Annie was in the public's eye more than before, she was still searching for a doctor to help with her speech problem.

Early one morning in 1992, her search came to an end. Her sister, Jane, was listening to the TV and heard this doctor tell about his school for people with speech problems.

Jane immediately thought of Annie and listened very intently to each word through the complete interview. She went immediately to the phone to call Annie. Jane wanted to relay the message that this doctor had told of his many, almost miraculous successes using his new methods of treatment.

Jane was unable to contact Annie that day, because Annie's phone was constantly busy.

P 36-38

The next day, when Jane finally got through, she found the reason that the phone was so busy was because the many friends Annie had throughout the whole country were trying to contact her also in hope that this doctor could help Annie.

In January of 1973, Annie attended Hollins College in Roanoke, Virginia, with much success. She practiced a great deal during these months. On Memorial Day, 1973, at Chagrin Falls, Ohio, in front of the Civil War Obelisk, Judge William Thomas introduced Annie to speak on behalf of her husband, who was speaking at another ceremony elsewhere. The judge was unaware this would be a first for her, but many people in the crowd knew of it.

Annie stood in silence for a few seconds and wondered if she could do it. She had never publicly made a speech before. With her usual courage and determination, Annie decided this would be a golden opportunity to try, and try she did.

The speech was such a success, that people who knew of her problem stood in tears. They knew what it meant to overcome this handicap that had plagued her all her life.

William Penn, the man who brought Annie's forefathers to America, brought to mind for Annie the first book he wrote during his religious persecution, "No Cross, No Glory."

P 39

It was a great victory for Annie that she had finally overcome her handicaps, one of the greatest being when she went into a store. Now there was no more feeling of frustration over clerks thinking her also deaf and not having to write everything down on paper.

P 40

Annie gets letters from people all over the world and answers all of them, helping in any way she can. She also gives an annual "Annie Glenn Award" for speech achievement.

P 41-42

Annie goes on to make speeches throughout many states, some are political and others are to speak about how she overcame her handicap. No one else was more elated over Annie's success in overcoming her problem than John. He had many agonizing thoughts about her handicap.

One morning, a young reporter found John sitting in tears in his office. The reporter asked John what was wrong, and John then proceeded to tell him that he was listening to Annie's very fluent tapes. He told the reporter that this relieved him of all the years of anxiety he had suffered.

Years later when John was being interviewed as one of the "Top Ten Persons of the Year" in America, he was asked who was the bravest person he ever knew, and without hesitating John replied, "Annie."

P 43

To handicapped children everywhere.
Let this story be an inspiration to sing out, "I shall overcome!"
Then you too will be able to sing, as Annie, "I have overcome!"

Annie

By B.P. Stetzel

JMJ

58498851R00032

Made in the USA
Lexington, KY
12 December 2016